PLANT-BASED CANCER DIET COOKBOOK

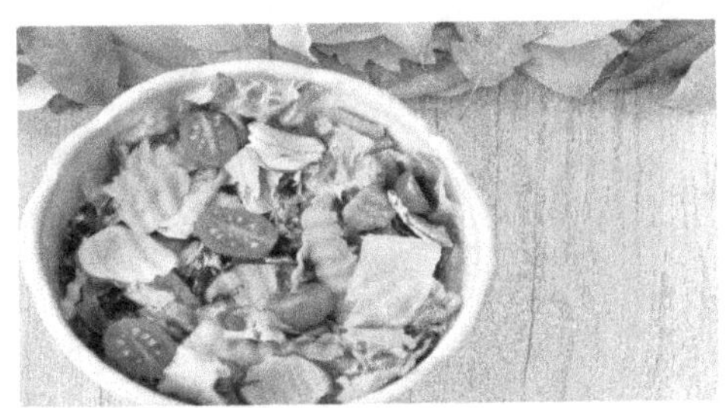

SUPER EASY AND TASTY PLANT-POWERED RECIPES TO REVERSE CANCER

MARIE HENDRICKS

Get the peppers ready: Turn the oven on to
375°F, or 190°C.Cut the bell peppers in half

creating plant-based staples like nut-based crusts, energy balls, and finely chopped veggies for salads or stir-fries. 92

3. Quality Knife Set: 92

A sharp and high-quality knife set is fundamental for precise and efficient cutting of fruits, vegetables, and herbs. Investing in good knives not only makes your cooking experience smoother but also ensures safety in the kitchen. 92

4. Steamer Basket: 92

Steaming is a gentle cooking method that helps retain the nutritional value of vegetables. A steamer basket is perfect for preparing a variety of plant-based ingredients, from broccoli and cauliflower to leafy greens and root vegetables. 92

5. Cast Iron Skillet: 92

A durable and versatile cast iron skillet is excellent for sautéing vegetables, making plant-based stir-fries, and even baking. It adds a depth of flavor to dishes and can go from stovetop to oven seamlessly. 93

6. Non-Stick Baking Sheets: 93

Baking sheets are essential for roasting a medley of vegetables or preparing plant-based snacks like kale chips. Opt for non-stick sheets to minimize the need for excessive oil. 93

7. Spiralizer: 93

A spiralizer is a fun tool that turns vegetables like zucchini, carrots, and sweet potatoes into noodle-like shapes. It's perfect for creating plant-based alternatives to traditional pasta dishes. 93

Whether you're creating vibrant salads, hearty soups, or innovative plant-based entrees, having the right kitchen equipment enhances efficiency and expands your culinary possibilities. As you embark on your plant-based cancer diet journey, invest in these tools to make the preparation of nourishing, flavorful meals an integral part of your Lifestyle 96

Start by planning your meals for the week. Identify simple and nutrient-dense recipes that align with a plant-based cancer diet. Include a variety of fruits, vegetables, whole grains, legumes, nuts, and seeds. Plan meals that are easy to prepare in larger quantities, making them suitable for batch cooking.   97

Invest in high-quality storage containers to keep your batch-cooked meals fresh. Consider batch cooking staples like grains (quinoa, brown rice), legumes (beans, lentils), and roasted vegetables. These can serve as the foundation for various dishes throughout the week.   98

Ensure variety in your batch-cooked meals to prevent monotony and provide a wide range of nutrients. Incorporate different colors, textures, and flavors into your dishes. Include cruciferous vegetables like broccoli and cauliflower, known for their potential cancer-fighting properties. 98

Explore plant-based protein sources such as

tofu, tempeh, edamame, and plant-based
protein powders. Incorporate these into your
batch-cooked meals to ensure you meet your
protein needs for the day. Protein is essential
for maintaining muscle mass and supporting
overall health.   98

6. Healthy Fats: 98

Include sources of healthy fats in your
batch-cooked meals, such as avocados, nuts,
seeds, and olive oil. These fats aid in satiety
and supply important fatty acids. In order to
keep your diet balanced, pay attention to
portion proportions.   98

7. Flavor Boosters: 98

Enhance the taste of your batch-cooked meals
with herbs, spices, and homemade sauces.
Experiment with different combinations to keep
your meals exciting and flavorful without relying
on excessive salt or sugar.   99

8. Efficient Cooking Techniques: 99

Optimize your time in the kitchen by using
efficient cooking techniques. Consider using a
slow cooker, Instant Pot, or sheet pan meals for
easy and time-saving preparation. These
methods allow you to cook large batches with
minimal effort.   99

9. Portion Control: 99

Divide your batch-cooked meals into
portion-controlled servings. This makes it easier
to grab a nutritious meal on busy days without
the need for additional preparation. Portion
control also helps prevent overeating.   99

10. Freeze for Convenience: 99

Label and date each container to track

freshness. Having a variety of frozen, pre-cooked meals provides convenience on days when cooking from scratch is not feasible. 100

In conclusion, batch cooking for busy days on a plant-based cancer diet involves thoughtful planning, diverse ingredient selection, and efficient cooking techniques. By incorporating these strategies into your routine, you can maintain a nourishing and cancer-conscious diet even during the most hectic days. Remember to stay flexible and enjoy the process of preparing wholesome meals that contribute to your overall well-being.

Servan-Schreiber, a physician and cancer survivor, explores lifestyle changes that can complement traditional cancer treatments. The book emphasizes the role of nutrition, stress management, and exercise in preventing and supporting cancer treatment.

5. "Radical Remission: Surviving Cancer Against All Odds" by Kelly A. Turner:

Turner explores cases of individuals who experienced unexpected recoveries from cancer. By studying these cases, she identifies commonalities in their approaches, providing hope and alternative perspectives on cancer treatment.

6. "Being Mortal: Medicine and What Matters in the End" by Atul Gawande:

While not exclusively about cancer, this book by surgeon Atul Gawande delves into the broader topic of end-of-life care. It offers valuable insights into the importance of quality of life, personal choices, and the human side of medical care, which can be particularly relevant for those dealing with cancer.

7. "Cancer: A Beginner's Guide" by Paul Scotting:

For those looking for a concise yet informative introduction to cancer, Scotting's book is a valuable resource. It covers the basics of cancer biology, treatment options, and emerging research in an accessible manner.

10. "My Sister's Keeper" by Jodi Picoult:

While a work of fiction, this novel explores the ethical and emotional complexities of dealing with cancer within a family. It raises thought-provoking questions about medical decisions, morality, and the impact of illness on relationships.   104

In conclusion, the recommended readings on cancer cover a broad spectrum, from scientific explorations to personal narratives and practical guides. These books collectively offer a well-rounded understanding of cancer, empowering individuals to make informed decisions, find support, and approach the journey with resilience and knowledge. Whether you are directly affected by cancer or seeking to educate yourself on the topic, these readings provide valuable insights into the multifaceted nature of this challenging diseases   104

**1. ** Information Sharing: 105

Online cancer communities serve as vast repositories of information. Members often share personal experiences with treatments, side effects, and coping strategies. This firsthand knowledge can be invaluable for someone newly diagnosed, offering practical insights that complement medical advice. From treatment options to lifestyle adjustments, the wealth of shared information fosters a sense of empowerment and informed decision-making. 105

2. Emotional Support: 105

Cancer can be an isolating experience, and online communities provide a virtual haven where individuals facing similar challenges can connect emotionally. Sharing fears, triumphs, and everyday struggles in a supportive environment helps reduce feelings of loneliness. Emotional support is a cornerstone of these communities, fostering a sense of belonging and understanding that transcends geographical boundaries.				105

One of the unique aspects of online cancer communities is the ability to connect with peers who have walked a similar path. Survivor stories inspire hope, and the empathy shared among those who have faced similar diagnoses or treatments can be deeply reassuring. These connections, often facilitated through forums, chat groups, or social media, create a supportive network that understands the nuances of the cancer journey.				105

Cancer doesn't only impact the individual diagnosed; it affects the entire support network, including caregivers. Online communities recognize the vital role caregivers play and provide dedicated spaces for them to share experiences, seek advice, and navigate the emotional challenges they face. Caregivers can connect with others who understand the unique demands of supporting a loved one through cancer treatment.				106

The immediacy of online platforms enables real-time communication, allowing community members to seek urgent advice, share updates, or simply vent when needed. Whether through instant messaging, video calls, or discussion forums, individuals can find timely support, fostering a sense of connection during critical moments in their cancer journey.				106

Many online cancer communities feature contributions from healthcare professionals, offering expert advice and clarifications on medical topics. While not a substitute for personalized medical consultation, these platforms provide a valuable additional resource for understanding treatment options, managing side effects, and staying informed about the latest advancements in cancer care. 106

Online cancer communities often compile and share a wealth of resources, including articles, webinars, and reputable information sources. This curated content covers a spectrum of topics, from practical tips on navigating insurance to emotional well-being and lifestyle adjustments. The collective knowledge within these communities transforms them into comprehensive libraries for individuals seeking guidance. 107

Beyond individual support, online cancer communities contribute to advocacy efforts and raise awareness about specific cancer types. Members often engage in discussions about research advancements, treatment options, and policy issues. This collective advocacy fosters a sense of purpose, as community members work together to raise awareness and improve outcomes for those affected by cancer. 107

The option for anonymity in online cancer communities allows individuals to share their experiences and concerns without revealing their identity. This can be particularly valuable for those who may feel uncomfortable discussing their diagnosis openly or wish to maintain privacy. The freedom to choose when and how much to disclose empowers individuals to engage at their own pace.   107

10. Long-Term Connections: 107

Online cancer communities can form enduring bonds among members. Shared experiences create a sense of camaraderie that extends beyond the initial stages of diagnosis and treatment. Members often celebrate milestones together, provide ongoing support during follow-up appointments, and continue to share insights as they transition into survivorship. 108

In conclusion, online communities and support networks have become integral components of the cancer journey, offering a virtual lifeline to those affected by the disease. Beyond information sharing, these platforms provide emotional support, foster peer connections, and contribute to advocacy efforts. As technology continues to advance, the role of online communities in cancer care is likely to evolve, providing even more opportunities for individuals to connect, learn, and navigate the complexities of their unique cancer journeys. 108

CONCLUSION   108

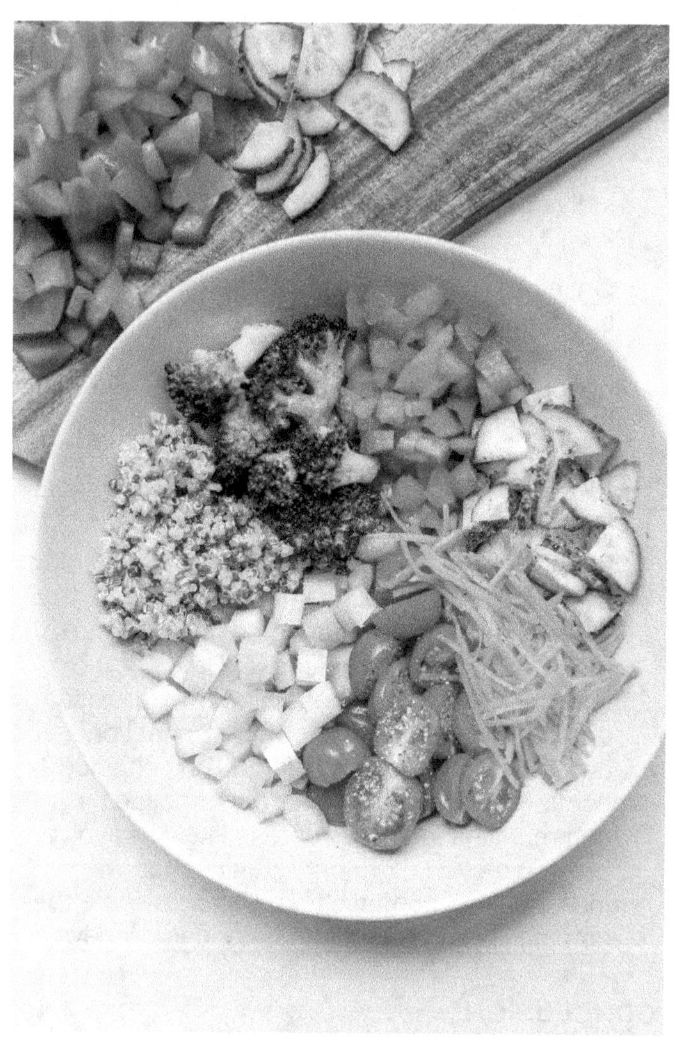

INTRODUCTION

Welcome to a culinary journey that goes beyond the ordinary—a journey fueled by the transformative power of a plant-based diet tailored for resilience against cancer. In these pages, we embark on a discovery of flavors, nutrients, and holistic well-being, crafting not just recipes but a lifestyle that nourishes and empowers.

In the face of the formidable challenge that cancer presents, we find hope in the vibrant spectrum of plant-based foods. This cookbook is not just a collection of recipes; it's a guide to harnessing the inherent healing potential within each ingredient. From nutrient-rich superfoods to comforting meals designed for strength, we invite you to explore a world where delicious meets nourishing, and every bite is a step towards vitality.

Whether you're on the path of prevention, in the midst of treatment, or embracing a post-cancer journey, this cookbook is your companion. Let's embark on a culinary adventure, embracing the bountiful offerings of the plant kingdom and, in doing so, cultivate a resilient spirit and a thriving, vibrant life. Here's to your health and the power of plants!

CHAPTER ONE

GETTING STARTED

- The Healing Power of Plant-Based Eating

In recent years, there has been a growing interest in the potential healing power of plant-based eating, particularly in its relation to cancer. As research continues to uncover the intricate links between nutrition and health, the role of a plant-based diet in preventing and managing cancer has become a subject of extensive investigation. This article explores the key aspects of how plant-based eating can positively impact individuals facing a cancer diagnosis.

The Foundation of Plant-Based Eating:

A plant-based diet is centered on whole, unprocessed plant foods, including fruits, vegetables, whole grains, legumes, nuts, and seeds. These foods are rich in essential nutrients, antioxidants, and phytochemicals, which collectively contribute to overall health and wellbeing. The emphasis on plant foods is characteristic of a diet that minimizes or eliminates animal products, avoiding red and processed meats, and reducing or eliminating dairy and eggs.

Cancer Prevention and Risk Reduction:

Numerous studies suggest that adopting a plant-based eating pattern may play a crucial role in preventing cancer and reducing the risk of its recurrence. The abundance of antioxidants and anti-inflammatory compounds found in plant foods helps combat oxidative stress and chronic inflammation, both of which are implicated in the development and progression of cancer.

Furthermore, a plant-based diet is often associated with a healthier body weight, and maintaining a healthy weight is a key factor in cancer prevention. Obesity is a known risk factor for various types of cancer, and the fiber-rich nature of plant-based foods contributes to satiety, making it easier for individuals to manage their weight.

Supporting Conventional Cancer Treatment:

While a plant-based diet is not a standalone cure for cancer, it can complement conventional cancer treatments such as surgery, chemotherapy, and radiation therapy. The nutritional density of plant foods ensures that individuals undergoing treatment receive vital nutrients necessary for maintaining strength and supporting the immune system.

Plant-based eating can also alleviate some of the side effects associated with cancer treatments. For instance, a diet rich in fruits and vegetables may help manage nausea, a common side effect of chemotherapy. Additionally, the anti-inflammatory properties of plant foods can contribute to reducing treatment-induced inflammation and promoting overall comfort.

Enhancing Immune Function:

The immune system plays a pivotal role in the body's defense against cancer cells. A plant-based diet, abundant in vitamins, minerals, and phytochemicals, supports and enhances immune function. Certain plant compounds, such as beta-glucans found in mushrooms and quercetin in onions, have been studied for their potential immune-boosting effects.

Moreover, the gut microbiota, influenced by diet, has emerged as a critical player in immune system regulation. Plant-based eating fosters a diverse and beneficial gut microbiome, which, in turn, positively impacts immune response and contributes to the body's ability to defend against cancer cells.

Managing Inflammation:

Chronic inflammation is a common denominator in various chronic diseases, including cancer.

Plant-based diets have been associated with anti-inflammatory effects, partly due to the presence of compounds like polyphenols and omega-3 fatty acids found in certain plant foods.

Reducing inflammation is particularly relevant in cancer prevention and treatment, as inflammation in the tumor microenvironment can contribute to tumor growth and progression. By adopting a plant-based eating pattern, individuals may mitigate inflammation, creating an environment less conducive to cancer development.

Conclusion:

The healing power of plant-based eating in the context of cancer is multifaceted. From cancer prevention and risk reduction to supporting conventional treatment and enhancing immune function, the benefits of a plant-based diet are increasingly recognized by the medical community. While it's essential to approach dietary changes as part of a comprehensive lifestyle strategy, the evidence suggests that plant-based eating can be a valuable ally in the fight against cancer, contributing to improved outcomes and a higher quality of life for individuals on their cancer journey

- ## Transitioning to a Plant-based Lifestyle

In the realm of cancer resilience, the power of lifestyle choices cannot be overstated. Amidst various approaches, transitioning to a plant-based diet emerges as a compelling and compassionate path. This shift is not merely about substituting animal products with plant alternatives; it's a holistic transformation that embraces the healing potential found in the diverse array of fruits, vegetables, grains, legumes, and nuts.

Embracing the Plant-Based Paradigm
The journey to a plant-based lifestyle is often marked by a paradigm shift—a reimagining of meals and a newfound appreciation for the bounty of nature. It's not just a dietary adjustment but a profound recognition of the impact our food choices can have on overall health, particularly in the context of cancer.

- ## The Healing Power of Plants

A plant-based diet is rich in phytochemicals, antioxidants, and fiber, which collectively contribute to a host of health benefits. These natural compounds found In fruits, vegetables, and whole grains have been shown to possess anti-inflammatory properties and play a role in cellular repair and regeneration—a crucial aspect in the fight against cancer.

- Reducing the Risk:
Plant-Based for Prevention
For those yet untouched by cancer, adopting a plant-based lifestyle can be a proactive measure to reduce the risk of developing certain types of cancer. Research indicates that diets abundant in plant foods are associated with a lower risk of cancer, potentially due to the protective effects of various phytonutrients.

- Supporting Treatment:
Plant-Based During Cancer Care
During cancer treatment, the body undergoes significant stress, and nutritional needs become paramount. A well-planned plant-based diet can offer a spectrum of nutrients essential for maintaining strength, managing side effects, and supporting the body's natural resilience. Plant foods are often easier to digest, aiding in the absorption of vital nutrients crucial for recovery.

Nourishing the Body and Soul
Beyond the physiological benefits, a plant-based lifestyle nourishes not only the body but also the soul. The vibrant colors, textures, and flavors present in plant-based meals create a culinary experience that is not only delicious but also emotionally satisfying. This connection between nourishment and well-being becomes a source of comfort and resilience, a crucial aspect of the cancer journey.

Practical Steps Toward a Plant-Based Life
Embarking on a plant-based journey may seem daunting initially, but a gradual and mindful approach can make the transition smoother and more sustainable. Here are some doable actions to help you:

1. Educate Yourself:
Understand the nutritional components of plant-based foods. Familiarize yourself with protein sources, essential vitamins, and minerals found in plants. This knowledge forms the foundation for crafting a balanced plant-based diet.

2. Start Gradually:
Transitioning doesn't have to be abrupt. Start by increasing the number of plant-based meals that you eat each day. Experiment with new recipes and gradually reduce reliance on animal products.

3. Diversify Your Plate:
Embrace variety. Explore a colorful array of fruits, vegetables, whole grains, legumes, nuts, and seeds. Diversifying your diet ensures a broad spectrum of nutrients.

4. Seek Support:
Connect with individuals who have embraced a plant-based lifestyle or join online communities. Sharing experiences and tips can provide invaluable support and motivation.

5. Consult with a Professional:
If you have specific dietary concerns or are undergoing cancer treatment, consult with a registered dietitian or healthcare professional. They can provide you with individualized advice based on your particular needs.

Embracing a Lifestyle of Resilience
Transitioning to a plant-based lifestyle is not a rigid set of rules but a dynamic journey of self-discovery. It's about savoring the flavors of health, nurturing your body with compassion, and cultivating resilience in the face of challenges.

As you embark on this transformative path, remember that small changes can yield profound results. Whether you're preventing cancer, undergoing treatment, or embracing life after cancer, a plant-based lifestyle can be a beacon of hope—a reminder that every bite is an opportunity to fuel your body with vitality and embrace a life of resilience and well-being.

- Stocking Your Plant-Powered Pantry

A well-stocked pantry is the foundation of a successful plant-based diet tailored for individuals facing cancer. Building a pantry filled with wholesome, nutrient-dense ingredients not only ensures that you have the essentials on hand but also contributes to a diet that may support overall well-being during cancer treatment. Let's delve into key components to consider when stocking your plant-powered pantry for a cancer-conscious approach.

1. Whole Grains:
Begin by selecting a variety of whole grains such as brown rice, quinoa, oats, and whole wheat pasta. These grains provide essential fiber, vitamins, and minerals, promoting digestive health and sustained energy levels – crucial factors during cancer treatment.

2. Legumes and Pulses:
Stock up on an assortment of legumes like lentils, chickpeas, black beans, and kidney beans. Rich in protein and fiber, legumes contribute to maintaining muscle mass and supporting digestive regularity, addressing common concerns during cancer therapy.

3. Healthy Fats:
Incorporate plant-based fats like extra virgin olive oil, avocados, and nuts. These sources of healthy fats offer a caloric boost, aid in nutrient absorption, and provide a satisfying element to meals, which can be particularly beneficial for individuals experiencing changes in appetite.

4. Nutrient-Packed Seeds:

Include seeds such as flaxseeds, chia seeds, and pumpkin seeds. These tiny powerhouses are loaded with omega-3 fatty acids, antioxidants, and essential minerals, contributing to heart health and overall nutritional support.

5. Herbs and Spices:
Enhance the flavor of your dishes with an array of herbs and spices. Turmeric, ginger, garlic, and cinnamon, known for their anti-inflammatory properties, can be valuable additions. Additionally, they can impart exciting flavors to meals, potentially making food more appealing for those undergoing taste alterations.

6. Cancer-Fighting Vegetables:
Opt for a rainbow of fresh and frozen vegetables. Dark leafy greens like kale and spinach, cruciferous vegetables such as broccoli and Brussels sprouts, and vibrant bell peppers offer a spectrum of vitamins, minerals, and antioxidants that may support the body's natural defense mechanisms.

7. Low-Sugar Fruits:
Choose low-sugar fruits like berries, apples, and citrus fruits. These fruits provide essential vitamins and antioxidants without causing spikes in blood sugar levels, which can be crucial for individuals managing side effects like fatigue and nausea.

8. Plant-Based Proteins:

Explore plant-based protein sources like tofu, tempeh, and plant-based protein powders. These options can assist in maintaining muscle mass and supporting the body's healing processes.

9. Whole Food Snacks:
Have wholesome snacks readily available. Air-popped popcorn, whole-grain crackers, and raw nuts make for satisfying snacks that can be easily incorporated into a cancer-conscious diet.

10. Hydration is Key:
Stock up on herbal teas, infused water, and coconut water to stay hydrated. Proper hydration is essential for overall health and well-being, especially during cancer treatment.

In conclusion, a thoughtfully stocked plant-powered pantry can play a pivotal role in supporting individuals navigating cancer treatment. By focusing on nutrient-dense, whole foods, you provide the body with the essential building blocks it needs for recovery and well-being. Tailoring the pantry to include a diverse range of foods ensures that you have the flexibility to create flavorful and nourishing meals, catering to individual tastes and nutritional needs during this challenging time

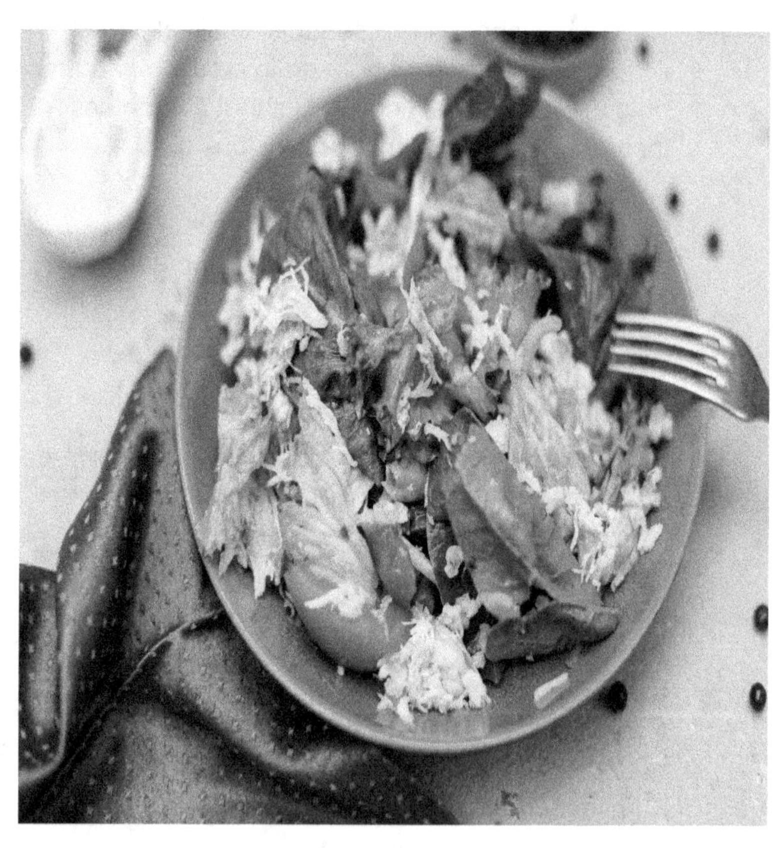

CHAPTER TWO

ESSENTIAL RECIPES FOR RESILIENCE

○ Perfect Smoothie Bowls

Anti-Cancer Smoothie Bowl Recipe
Ingredients:
Base:

1 cup frozen mixed berries (blueberries, raspberries, and strawberries)
1 banana (ripe)
1/2 cup Greek yogurt (unsweetened)
1/4 cup almond milk (unsweetened)
Toppings:

2 tablespoons chia seeds (rich in omega-3 fatty acids)
1 tablespoon flaxseeds (contain lignans, which may have protective effects)
1/4 cup walnuts (source of antioxidants and omega-3 fatty acids)
1/2 cup fresh kiwi slices (packed with vitamin C)
1/4 cup pomegranate seeds (contain antioxidants)
Optional Add-ins:

1 teaspoon turmeric powder (known for its anti-inflammatory properties)
1 teaspoon spirulina (a nutrient-rich algae with potential health benefits)
Instructions:
Blend the Base:

In a blender, combine the frozen berries, banana, Greek yogurt, and almond milk.
Blend until smooth and creamy.
Prepare Toppings:

Slice fresh kiwi and gather the walnuts, chia seeds, flaxseeds, and pomegranate seeds.
Assemble the Bowl:

Pour the smoothie into a bowl.
Add Toppings:

Arrange the kiwi slices, sprinkle chia seeds, flaxseeds, and pomegranate seeds on top.
Crush the walnuts and spread them over the bowl.
Optional Enhancements:

If desired, sprinkle turmeric powder for added anti-inflammatory benefits.
Consider adding spirulina for an extra nutrient boost.

Serve and Enjoy:

Enjoy your delicious and nutrient-packed anti-cancer smoothie bowl!
Remember, a diet rich in fruits, vegetables, and nuts may contribute to overall health, including potential cancer-fighting properties. However, it's essential to consult with a healthcare professional for personalized advice and treatment regarding cancer or any health condition.

o   Nourishing Buddha Bowls

In the realm of cancer prevention and overall well-being, dietary choices play a pivotal role. One culinary trend that aligns seamlessly with these health goals is the Nourishing Buddha Bowl. These bowls not only provide a delightful sensory experience but are also packed with a plethora of nutrients that have been associated with potential cancer-fighting properties.

Components of a Cancer-Fighting Buddha Bowl:
1. Base Grains:
Start your Buddha Bowl with a foundation of whole grains. Brown rice, quinoa, or farro can be excellent choices. Whole grains are rich in fiber, which has been linked to a reduced risk of certain cancers. The

fiber content aids in digestion and helps maintain a healthy weight, a factor crucial in cancer prevention.

2. Abundance of Colorful Vegetables:
Incorporate a vibrant array of vegetables into your bowl. Broccoli, kale, spinach, carrots, and bell peppers are not only visually appealing but are also packed with antioxidants. These compounds combat free radicals in the body, potentially reducing the risk of cellular damage that could lead to cancer.

3. Lean Proteins:
Choose lean protein sources like grilled chicken, tofu, or legumes such as chickpeas and lentils. These proteins are essential for muscle maintenance and repair while offering an alternative to red and processed meats, which are linked to an increased risk of certain cancers.

4. Healthy Fats:
Incorporate foods like avocados, almonds, and seeds that are good sources of fat. Avocados in particular, are rich in monounsaturated fats, which have been associated with a decreased risk of breast cancer. Nuts and seeds, such as flaxseeds and chia seeds, contribute omega-3 fatty acids, known for their anti-inflammatory properties.

5. Antioxidant-Rich Dressings:
Opt for homemade dressings using olive oil, garlic, and herbs. Olive oil, a staple in the Mediterranean diet, contains polyphenols that possess antioxidant and anti-inflammatory properties. Garlic, part of the

allium vegetable family, has shown potential in inhibiting cancer cell growth.

The Science Behind Buddha Bowls and Cancer Prevention:
1. Anti-Inflammatory Benefits:
The ingredients commonly found in Buddha Bowls, such as leafy greens, berries, and turmeric, are known for their anti-inflammatory properties. Chronic inflammation is linked to the development of cancer, and incorporating anti-inflammatory foods can be a proactive measure in reducing this risk.

2. Regulation of Blood Sugar Levels:
Whole grains and fiber-rich vegetables help regulate blood sugar levels. Maintaining stable blood sugar is crucial, as elevated levels have been associated with an increased risk of various cancers.

3. Phytochemical Powerhouses:
The diverse range of vegetables and fruits in Buddha Bowls provides an abundance of phytochemicals. These natural compounds have demonstrated potential anticancer effects by interfering with processes that promote the growth of cancer cells.

Practical Tips for Creating Cancer-Fighting Buddha Bowls:
Diversity Matters: Aim for a colorful mix of vegetables to ensure a broad spectrum of nutrients.

Portion Control: While Buddha Bowls are nutrient-dense, maintaining appropriate portion sizes is crucial for overall health.

Hydration is Key: Pair your Buddha Bowl with water or herbal teas to stay adequately hydrated, another essential aspect of cancer prevention.

Cancer-Fighting Buddha Bowl Recipes:
1. Mediterranean Inspired Bowl:
Ingredients:
1 cup cooked quinoa
1 cup cherry tomatoes, halved
1/2 cucumber, diced
1/4 cup Kalamata olives, sliced
1/4 cup feta cheese, crumbled
Grilled chicken breast (optional)
Instructions:
Assemble quinoa as the base.
Arrange tomatoes, cucumber, olives, and feta.
Add grilled chicken if desired.
Season with oregano and a drizzle of olive oil.

2. Plant-Powered Protein Bowl:
Ingredients:
1 cup cooked brown rice
1 cup mixed greens (kale, spinach)
1/2 cup cooked chickpeas
1/4 cup avocado, sliced
2 tablespoons pumpkin seeds
Tahini dressing
Instructions:
Place brown rice as the base.

Top with mixed greens, chickpeas, and avocado.
Sprinkle pumpkin seeds.
Drizzle with tahini dressing.
These recipes provide a delicious way to incorporate cancer-fighting ingredients into your diet. Remember to adapt based on personal preferences and consult with healthcare professionals for personalized advice, especially if you have specific health concerns or conditions like cancer. The information provided here serves as general guidance and is not a substitute for professional medical advice

○ **Anti-Inflammatory Turmeric Soup**

turmeric has gained acclaim for its potent anti-inflammatory properties, with studies suggesting potential benefits in cancer prevention and treatment. Harnessing the power of this golden spice, we present a comforting and nutrient-packed Anti-Inflammatory Turmeric Soup that not only tantalizes the taste buds but also promotes overall well-being.

Ingredients:
1 tablespoon olive oil
1 onion, finely chopped
3 cloves garlic, minced
1 tablespoon fresh ginger, grated
1 teaspoon ground turmeric
1 teaspoon ground cumin
1 teaspoon ground coriander
1 cup carrots, diced

1 cup sweet potatoes, diced
1 cup cauliflower florets
4 cups vegetable broth
1 cup coconut milk
Salt and pepper to taste
Fresh cilantro for garnish
Instructions:
Saute Aromatics:
In a big saucepan, warm up the olive oil over medium heat.
 Add finely chopped onions, minced garlic, and grated ginger. Saute until the onions are translucent and aromatic.

Spice Infusion:
Sprinkle ground turmeric, cumin, and coriander over the sauteed aromatics. Stir well to coat the vegetables in these flavorful spices, enhancing both taste and health benefits.

Vegetable Medley:
Add diced carrots, sweet potatoes, and cauliflower florets to the pot. These colorful vegetables not only lend a vibrant hue to the soup but also contribute essential vitamins and minerals.

Golden Elixir:
Pour in vegetable broth, creating a nourishing base for the soup. The combination of turmeric and broth forms a golden elixir, rich in anti-inflammatory compounds that may aid in cancer prevention.

Simmer to Perfection:

Allow the soup to simmer gently, letting the flavors meld together. This slow cooking process enhances the infusion of turmeric and spices into the broth, ensuring a robust and comforting flavor profile.

Creamy Indulgence:
Pour in coconut milk, adding a creamy and luscious texture to the soup. Coconut milk not only complements the earthy notes of turmeric but also brings healthy fats to the mix.

Season to Taste:
To taste, adjust the amount of salt and pepper used to season the soup.
Adjusting the seasoning ensures a personalized touch to suit individual taste buds.

Garnish and Serve:
Ladle the golden soup into bowls, garnishing with fresh cilantro for a burst of freshness. Cilantro not only adds a delightful aroma but also contributes additional anti-inflammatory properties.

Conclusion:
This Anti-Inflammatory Turmeric Soup is not just a culinary delight; it's a nourishing bowl of wellness. Packed with antioxidants and anti-inflammatory compounds, each spoonful may offer potential benefits in the journey towards cancer prevention and overall health. Embrace the warmth of this healing soup and savor the goodness that nature provides.

○ Quinoa and Roasted Veggie Power Bowl

In the realm of cancer-fighting cuisine, the Quinoa and Roasted Veggie Power Bowl stands out as a nutritional powerhouse. This vibrant and nourishing dish not only brings a burst of flavors to the table but also packs a punch in terms of health benefits.

Ingredients:

1 cup quinoa, rinsed
2 cups mixed vegetables (such as broccoli, bell peppers, carrots), chopped
1 tablespoon olive oil
1 teaspoon garlic powder
1 teaspoon dried oregano
Salt and pepper to taste
Instructions:

- Preheat and Prepare:
Start by preheating your oven to 400°F (200°C). Meanwhile, rinse the quinoa thoroughly under cold water to remove any bitterness.

Cook Quinoa:
In a medium saucepan, combine the rinsed quinoa with 2 cups of water. Bring to a boil, then reduce heat, cover, and simmer for about 15 minutes or until the quinoa is cooked and water is absorbed.

- Prepare Vegetables:

While the quinoa is cooking, toss the chopped vegetables in olive oil, garlic powder, dried oregano, salt, and pepper.Arrange them uniformly on a baking tray.

- Roast Vegetables:
  Roast the seasoned vegetables in the preheated oven for 20-25 minutes or until they are tender and slightly caramelized, stirring halfway through for even cooking.

- Assemble the Power Bowl:
Once the quinoa and roasted veggies are ready, assemble your power bowl. Start with a generous scoop of quinoa as the base, then top it with the flavorful roasted vegetables.

- Customize and Garnish:
Feel free to customize your bowl by adding extras like avocado slices, a sprinkle of nutritional yeast, or a drizzle of tahini for added creaminess and flavor.

- Health Benefits:
 This Quinoa and Roasted Veggie Power Bowl is not only a delight for your taste buds but also a nutritional ally in the fight against cancer. Quinoa, a complete protein, provides essential amino acids crucial for cellular repair and regeneration. The colorful assortment of vegetables brings a spectrum of vitamins, minerals, and antioxidants, supporting overall well-being and a robust immune system.

Conclusion: Embrace the wholesome goodness of this Quinoa and Roasted Veggie Power Bowl as a delicious addition to your cancer-fighting culinary arsenal. Its combination of nutrient-dense ingredients not only satisfies your palate but contributes to a balanced and health-conscious lifestyle.

Incorporating such vibrant and nutrient-packed recipes into your plant-based diet cookbook can contribute significantly to the holistic well-being of those navigating the challenges of cancer.

CHAPTER THREE

HEALING MAINS

- ○ Lentil and Mushroom Stuffed Peppers

Ingredients:

Four big bell peppers, seeded and halved

1 cup green or brown lentils, cooked
1 cup mushrooms, finely chopped
1 onion, finely diced
2 cloves garlic, minced
1 cup spinach, chopped
1 teaspoon cumin
1 teaspoon paprika
Salt and pepper to taste
1 can (14 oz) crushed tomatoes
1 cup vegetable broth
1 cup cooked quinoa (optional)
Fresh parsley for garnish

Instructions:
Get the peppers ready: Turn the oven on to 375°F, or
190°C.Cut the bell peppers in half lengthwise and
remove the seeds and membranes. Place them in a
baking dish.

Saute Vegetables:
In a large skillet, sauté the onions and garlic until they
become translucent. Add the finely chopped
mushrooms and cook until they release their moisture
and become golden brown.

Add Lentils and Spinach:
 Incorporate the cooked lentils into the skillet, followed
by the chopped spinach. Stir in the cumin, paprika,
salt, and pepper, allowing the flavors to meld together.

Combine with Tomatoes and Broth:

Pour in the crushed tomatoes and vegetable broth, creating a savory and rich base for the stuffing. Allow the mixture to simmer for about 10 minutes, letting the flavors intensify.

Fill the Peppers:
 Spoon the lentil and mushroom mixture into each halved bell pepper, ensuring they are generously filled. If desired, mix in cooked quinoa for an additional layer of texture and nutritional value.

To achieve the perfect bake, place aluminum foil over the baking dish and bake it in a preheated oven for a duration of 25-30 minutes.This gentle cooking process allows the peppers to become tender and absorb the savory essence of the stuffing.

Garnish and Serve: Once out of the oven, garnish the stuffed peppers with fresh parsley for a burst of color and added freshness. Serve them hot, creating a visually appealing and incredibly satisfying dish.

Healing Properties: The Lentil and Mushroom Stuffed Peppers not only captivate the taste buds but also deliver a plethora of healing benefits. Lentils, rich in protein and fiber, support digestive health and provide a steady release of energy. Mushrooms contribute immune-boosting properties and add a savory depth to the dish. The colorful bell peppers bring a wealth of antioxidants, essential for neutralizing free radicals in the body.

Conclusion: Including the Lentil and Mushroom Stuffed Peppers in your cancer diet cookbook is a testament to the fusion of delicious flavors and healing properties. This nutrient-packed main not only satiates the appetite but also serves as a testament to the potential of plant-based cuisine in promoting overall well-being, especially for those on a cancer-fighting journey.

○ **Chickpea and Spinach Curry**

Chickpea and Spinach Curry is a delightful vegetarian dish that marries the robust flavors of chickpeas with the vibrant goodness of spinach. This nutrient-rich curry not only pleases the palate but also provides a wholesome meal packed with protein, fiber, and essential vitamins. Here's a comprehensive guide to crafting this delectable dish:

Ingredients:
Two 15-ounce cans of rinsed and drained chickpeas each

1 large onion, finely chopped
3 cloves garlic, minced
1-inch piece of ginger, grated
2 cups fresh spinach, washed and chopped
One fourteen-ounce can of diced tomatoes or two big
tomatoes chopped
1 can (14 oz) coconut milk
2 tablespoons cooking oil
1 teaspoon cumin seeds
1 teaspoon ground coriander
1 teaspoon turmeric powder
1 teaspoon garam masala
Half a teaspoon red chili powder, or more according to
taste
Salt to taste
Fresh cilantro for garnish
Instructions:

Sauté Aromatics:
In a big pan, warm up the oil over medium heat.
Sprinkle in the cumin seeds and watch them pop.
Chop the onions and cook them until they get golden
brown.
Add the grated ginger and minced garlic, and cook for
an additional minute.
Create the Spice Base:

Lower the heat and add ground coriander, turmeric,
garam masala, and red chili powder.
Stir well to create a fragrant spice base.
Introduce Chickpeas:

Add drained and rinsed chickpeas to the pan.

Ensure the chickpeas are well-coated with the aromatic spice blend.
Allow them to cook for 5-7 minutes, absorbing the flavors.
Incorporate Tomatoes:

Pour in the diced tomatoes or fresh chopped tomatoes.
Cook until the tomatoes break down and release their juices, forming a rich base.
Wilt in Spinach:

Add the chopped spinach to the pan.
Allow the spinach to wilt and cook down, imparting its vibrant color and nutritional goodness.
Creamy Consistency:

Pour in the coconut milk to add a creamy consistency to the curry.
Stir well and let the flavors meld for an additional 5-7 minutes.

Season to Perfection:
Add salt to taste while seasoning the curry.
You can add extra red chili powder if you'd like it hotter.

Garnish and Serve:
Sprinkle some fresh cilantro on top of the chickpea and spinach curry.
Accompany it with warm naan bread or on a bed of fluffy basmati rice.

Tips for Perfection:
Spice amounts: Change the amounts of spice to suit your taste.
 Feel free to add more or less chili powder based on your taste.

Creaminess: For a richer curry, you can use full-fat coconut milk.
 Use light coconut milk if you would want it be lighter. Variations: Experiment with additional vegetables like bell peppers or peas to add more color and texture.

Meal Prep: This curry freezes well, making it an excellent option for meal prepping.For later usage, keep it sealed in containers.

Chickpea and Spinach Curry is a versatile dish that caters to both flavor enthusiasts and health-conscious individuals. Its simplicity in preparation, coupled with the rich blend of spices and nutritious ingredients, makes it a go-to recipe for those seeking a hearty and satisfying vegetarian meal. Whether you're a seasoned chef or a novice in the kitchen, this curry promises a culinary adventure that tantalizes the taste buds and nourishes the body.

Grilled Portobello Mushrooms with Herbed Quinoa

Grilled Portobello Mushrooms with Herbed Quinoa is a wholesome and flavorful dish that not only tantalizes the taste buds but also incorporates ingredients with potential health benefits, especially in the context of cancer. Let's explore the key components and their potential contributions.

Grilled Portobello Mushrooms:
Portobello mushrooms are a nutritional powerhouse. They are rich in antioxidants, including selenium, which may have cancer-fighting properties. Additionally, mushrooms contain beta-glucans, compounds that can modulate the immune system. The grilling process enhances their savory flavor and imparts a delightful smokiness.

Recipe:

Ingredients:

Portobello mushrooms
Olive oil
Garlic powder
Salt and pepper
Balsamic vinegar (optional)
Instructions:
a. Clean the mushrooms and remove the stems.
b. Mix olive oil, garlic powder, salt, and pepper to create a marinade.
c. Brush the mushrooms with the marinade.
d. Grill for about 5-7 minutes on each side until they are tender.
e. Optionally, drizzle with balsamic vinegar before serving.

Herbed Quinoa:
Quinoa is a versatile whole grain that provides a good
source of protein, fiber, and various essential
nutrients. It contains quercetin, a flavonoid with
potential anti-cancer properties, and its high fiber
content supports digestive health.

Recipe:

Ingredients:

Quinoa
Vegetable broth
Herbs that are fresh, like parsley, thyme, or rosemary
Lemon juice
Salt and pepper
Instructions:
a. Rinse quinoa under cold water.
b. Cook quinoa in vegetable broth for added flavor.
c. Fluff cooked quinoa with a fork.
d. Add finely chopped fresh herbs, lemon juice, salt,
and pepper to taste.

Assembly:
Combine the grilled Portobello mushrooms with the
herbed quinoa for a dish that balances the earthy
richness of the mushrooms with the lightness of the
quinoa. The result is a satisfying and nutritious meal
that can be a valuable addition to a plant-based diet.

Health Considerations:

Antioxidants: The combination of antioxidants from both mushrooms and quinoa may help combat oxidative stress, a factor linked to cancer development.
Fiber Content: High fiber intake is associated with a lower risk of certain cancers, and quinoa contributes to achieving recommended daily fiber goals.
Plant-Based Proteins: Both mushrooms and quinoa offer plant-based protein, supporting muscle health without the potential drawbacks of animal-based proteins.
In conclusion, Grilled Portobello Mushrooms with Herbed Quinoa is a delightful and nutritionally dense dish that aligns with a plant-based approach to cancer prevention. Incorporating such recipes into a balanced diet can contribute to overall health and well-being.

CHAPTER FOUR

SNACKS AND SWEETS

○   Nutty Energy Bites

A plant-based diet rich in fruits, vegetables, whole grains, and nuts has been associated with a reduced risk of certain cancers and improved overall well-being. Nutty Energy Bites, a delightful and convenient snack, can be a flavorful addition to this cancer-fighting approach, providing essential nutrients and satisfying cravings while aligning with a plant-based lifestyle.

Plant-Based Diets' Potential to Prevent Cancer. Numerous studies suggest that plant-based diets may help prevent cancer and support those undergoing cancer treatment. These diets are typically abundant in antioxidants, vitamins, minerals, and phytochemicals, all of which play crucial roles in maintaining a healthy immune system and reducing inflammation – factors that are closely linked to cancer development.

The Role of Nuts in Cancer-Fighting Nutrition Nuts, a key ingredient in Nutty Energy Bites, are nutritional powerhouses known for their rich content of healthy fats, protein, fiber, vitamins, and minerals. They also contain antioxidants, such as vitamin E and selenium, which contribute to the neutralization of free radicals in the body, potentially reducing the risk of cellular damage that can lead to cancer.

Nutty Energy Bites: A Cancer-Fighting Snack
Ingredients:
1 cup rolled oats
1/2 cup nut butter (almond, peanut, or cashew)
1/3 cup honey or maple syrup
1/2 cup ground flaxseeds
1/4 cup of finely chopped nuts (almonds, pistachios, or walnuts)
1/3 cup dark chocolate chips (optional)
1 teaspoon vanilla extract
A pinch of salt
Instructions:
Combine Dry Ingredients: In a mixing bowl, combine rolled oats, ground flaxseeds, chopped nuts, and a pinch of salt.
To make sure the components are distributed evenly, thoroughly mix.
Add Wet Ingredients: Incorporate the nut butter, honey or maple syrup, and vanilla extract into the dry mixture. Stir until the ingredients are well combined and form a cohesive mixture.

Fold in Chocolate Chips (Optional): For an extra touch of sweetness, fold in dark chocolate chips. This step is optional but adds a delightful burst of flavor.

Form Bite-Sized Balls: Take small portions of the mixture and roll them into bite-sized balls using your hands. The size can be adjusted based on personal preference.

Chill and Serve: Place the energy bites on a tray lined with parchment paper and let them chill in the refrigerator for at least 30 minutes. Once firm, these Nutty Energy Bites are ready to be enjoyed.

Nutrient Highlights:
Omega-3 Fatty Acids: Flaxseeds contribute omega-3 fatty acids, which have anti-inflammatory properties that may aid in cancer prevention.

Fiber: Oats and flaxseeds are excellent sources of fiber, promoting digestive health and assisting in the elimination of toxins.

Protein: Nuts and nut butter provide a plant-based protein source, crucial for maintaining muscle mass and supporting overall bodily functions.

Antioxidants: The combination of nuts and dark chocolate chips introduces antioxidants that combat oxidative stress, a contributing factor to cancer development.

Incorporating Nutty Energy Bites into a plant-based diet not only enhances nutritional intake but also offers a delightful and convenient snack option. These bites are not only delicious but also align with the principles of a cancer-fighting diet by providing a balance of essential nutrients. Remember that while diet plays a crucial role in overall health, it's essential to consult with healthcare professionals for personalized advice, especially in the context of cancer prevention and treatment.

○ Avocado Chocolate Mousse

Avocados, a key ingredient in this delectable mousse, are rich in monounsaturated fats and contain various bioactive compounds. These compounds, including carotenoids and tocopherols, exhibit antioxidant properties that help neutralize free radicals in the body. Free radicals can contribute to the development of cancer by damaging cellular DNA.

Additionally, avocados provide a good source of fiber, promoting digestive health and aiding in the elimination of toxins from the body. This fiber-rich content supports a healthy gut microbiome, which has been linked to a reduced risk of certain cancers.

The Role of Dark Chocolate in a Cancer-Fighting Diet Dark chocolate, the second star of this dessert, is known for its high concentration of flavonoids. Flavonoids, with their antioxidant and anti-inflammatory properties, contribute to cellular health and may help prevent cancer development. Moreover, dark chocolate contains theobromine, a compound that has been studied for its potential anti-cancer effects.

Avocado Chocolate Mousse Recipe
Ingredients:
2 ripe avocados

1/2 cup unsweetened cocoa powder
1/2 cup maple syrup or agave nectar
1/3 cup almond milk (or any plant-based milk)
1 teaspoon vanilla extract
A pinch of salt
Dark chocolate shavings (for garnish)
Instructions:
Prepare the Avocados:

Cut the avocados in half, remove the pits, and scoop
out the flesh into a blender or food processor.
Blend Ingredients:

Add cocoa powder, maple syrup (or agave nectar),
almond milk, vanilla extract, and a pinch of salt to the
blender.
Blend Until Smooth:

Blend the ingredients until the mixture becomes
smooth and creamy.
To make sure there is even mixing, scrape down the
sides of the blender.

Adjust Sweetness:
Taste the mousse and adjust the sweetness if needed
by adding more maple syrup or agave nectar.
Chill:

Transfer the mousse into serving glasses or bowls
and refrigerate for at least 2 hours, allowing it to set
and intensify the flavors.
Garnish and Serve:

Before serving, garnish with dark chocolate shavings for an extra touch of indulgence.
Conclusion
Indulging in a decadent dessert like Avocado Chocolate Mousse doesn't mean compromising on health, especially when it aligns with the principles of a plant-based cancer-fighting diet. By incorporating nutrient-dense ingredients such as avocados and dark chocolate, you not only satisfy your sweet tooth but also provide your body with powerful antioxidants and anti-inflammatory compounds. This delicious dessert proves that healthy eating can be both enjoyable

○ **Roasted Chickpeas Three Ways**

In the quest for a health-conscious lifestyle, incorporating nutrient-dense foods with potential cancer-fighting properties has become a focal point. Roasted chickpeas, a versatile and delicious snack, emerge as a powerhouse in this regard. Packed with fiber, protein, and an array of essential nutrients, chickpeas offer a foundation for creating cancer-fighting snacks that not only satisfy the taste buds but also contribute to overall well-being.

1. The Nutritional Arsenal of Chickpeas:
Chickpeas, also known as garbanzo beans, are a nutrient-rich legume celebrated for their high fiber content, providing a sense of satiety while aiding in digestive health. Rich in plant-based protein, chickpeas supply the body with essential amino acids necessary for cell repair and regeneration. Moreover, they are a source of key vitamins and minerals,

including folate, iron, phosphorus, and manganese, each playing a role in supporting various bodily functions.

2. The Cancer-Fighting Potential:
Research suggests that certain compounds found in chickpeas may have cancer-fighting properties. For instance, the presence of saponins, a type of plant compound, has been associated with anti-cancer effects. Additionally, chickpeas contain antioxidants, such as quercetin and chlorogenic acid, which combat oxidative stress and inflammation – both factors linked to cancer development.

3. Roasting Magic Unveiled:
Roasting chickpeas not only enhances their natural nutty flavor but also transforms them into a crunchy, satisfying snack. The three variations presented here incorporate cancer-fighting ingredients, elevating the nutritional profile while maintaining a delightful taste.

a. Turmeric and Black Pepper Infusion:
Ingredients:

2 cans of chickpeas, drained and rinsed
1 teaspoon turmeric
1/2 teaspoon black pepper
2 tablespoons olive oil
Pinch of sea salt
Instructions:

Preheat the oven to 400°F (200°C).

In a bowl, combine chickpeas, turmeric, black pepper,
olive oil, and sea salt. Toss until chickpeas are
well-coated.
Arrange the chickpeas in a single layer on a baking
sheet.
Roast for 25-30 minutes or until golden brown and
crunchy, stirring halfway through.
b. Garlic and Rosemary Elegance:
Ingredients:

2 cans of chickpeas, drained and rinsed
3 cloves garlic, minced
2 tablespoons fresh rosemary, finely chopped
2 tablespoons olive oil
Dash of cayenne pepper (optional)
Instructions:

Preheat the oven to 400°F (200°C).
In a bowl, combine chickpeas, minced garlic,
rosemary, olive oil, and cayenne pepper. Toss until
chickpeas are evenly coated.
On a baking sheet, distribute the chickpeas in a single
layer.
Roast, tossing halfway through, for 25 to 30 minutes,
or until crispy.

c. Cumin and Paprika Fiesta:
Ingredients:

2 cans of chickpeas, drained and rinsed
1 teaspoon ground cumin
1 teaspoon paprika
2 tablespoons olive oil

Sprinkle of nutritional yeast
Instructions:

Preheat the oven to 400°F (200°C).
In a bowl, combine chickpeas, cumin, paprika, olive oil, and nutritional yeast. Toss until chickpeas are well-coated.
In a single layer, distribute the chickpeas on a baking sheet.
Roast for 25-30 minutes or until golden and crunchy, stirring halfway through.

4. Incorporating Roasted Chickpeas into a Balanced Diet:
While these roasted chickpea variations offer cancer-fighting potential, it's crucial to view them as part of a well-rounded, plant-based diet. Including a variety of colorful fruits and vegetables, whole grains, and lean proteins complements the benefits of roasted chickpeas, contributing to overall health and reducing the risk of cancer.

5. Conclusion:
A Culinary Journey Towards Health:
Incorporating roasted chickpeas three ways into one's diet not only introduces a delicious and crunchy snack but also leverages the potential cancer-fighting properties of this humble legume. Embracing a diet rich in nutrient-dense foods, such as chickpeas, aligns with a proactive approach to health, offering a tasty and satisfying way to support the body's natural defense mechanisms against cancer.

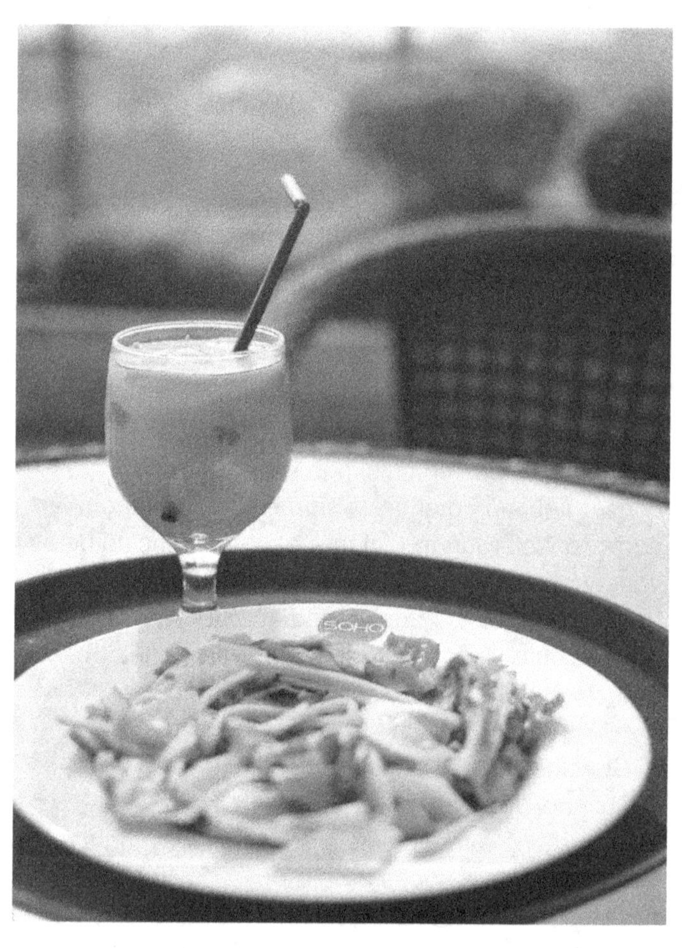

CHAPTER FIVE

MEAL PLANS FOR EVERY WEEK

○ One-Week Kickstart Plan

Ingredients:

2 cups kale
1 cup spinach
1 ripe banana
1/2 cup mixed berries
1 cup almond milk or water
Instructions:

Blend kale, spinach, banana, and mixed berries with almond milk or water until smooth.
Pour into a glass and enjoy the nutrient-packed start to your day.
Lunch: Quinoa and Veggie Delight

Ingredients:

1 cup quinoa, cooked
1 cup mixed vegetables (bell peppers, cucumber, cherry tomatoes)
Lemon-tahini dressing
Instructions:

Cook quinoa according to package instructions.
Mix cooked quinoa with chopped vegetables.
Drizzle with lemon-tahini dressing for a flavorful and satisfying lunch.

Dinner: Hearty Lentil and Vegetable Stew

Ingredients:
1 cup dried lentils, rinsed
2 carrots, diced
2 celery stalks, chopped
1 onion, diced
4 cups vegetable broth
Spices (cumin, coriander, paprika)
Instructions:
In a pot, combine lentils, carrots, celery, onion, and
vegetable broth.
Add spices to taste and simmer until lentils
are tender.
Serve warm for a filling and healthy supper.

Day 2: Cruciferous Crusade
Breakfast: Broccoli and Avocado Toast with Pumpkin
Seeds

Ingredients:

2 slices whole-grain bread
1 ripe avocado
1 cup broccoli florets, steamed
2 tbsp pumpkin seeds
Instructions:

Toast the bread slices.
Mash avocado and spread it on the toast.
Top with steamed broccoli and sprinkle with pumpkin
seeds.
Lunch: Cauliflower and Chickpea Curry

Ingredients:

1 small cauliflower, chopped
1 can chickpeas, drained
1 can coconut milk
Curry spices (turmeric, cumin, coriander)
2 cups cooked whole-grain rice
Instructions:

In a pot, combine cauliflower, chickpeas, coconut
milk, and curry spices.
Simmer until cauliflower is tender.
Serve over cooked whole-grain rice for a satisfying
lunch.
Dinner: Roasted Brussels Sprouts and Sweet Potato
Bowl with Balsamic Glaze

Ingredients:

2 cups Brussels sprouts, halved
1 large sweet potato, diced
2 tbsp olive oil
Balsamic glaze
Instructions:
Mix sweet potato and Brussels sprouts together with
olive oil.
Roast in the oven until golden and crispy.
Drizzle with balsamic glaze before serving.
Day 3: Berry Boost
Breakfast: Mixed Berry Chia Pudding

Ingredients:

1/4 cup chia seeds
1 cup almond milk
Mixed berries (strawberries, blueberries, raspberries)

Instructions:
Stir the chia seeds into the almond milk and
refrigerate for the entire night.
In the morning, top with a variety of fresh berries for a
burst of antioxidants.
Lunch: Kale and Berry Salad with Walnuts and Citrus
Vinaigrette

Ingredients:

2 cups kale, chopped
Mixed berries
1/4 cup walnuts, chopped
Citrus vinaigrette
Instructions:

Toss chopped kale with mixed berries and walnuts.
Drizzle with citrus vinaigrette for a refreshing and
nutritious salad.
Dinner: Blueberry and Almond Crusted Tofu

Ingredients:

1 block extra-firm tofu, pressed and sliced
1/2 cup blueberries
1/4 cup almonds, crushed
Maple syrup for drizzling
Instructions:

Coat tofu slices with crushed almonds and
blueberries.
After baking till golden, pour with maple syrup and
serve.

Day 4: Rainbow Delight
Breakfast: Rainbow Fruit Bowl

Ingredients:

Assorted colorful fruits (strawberries, kiwi, pineapple,
mango, blueberries)
Instructions:

Slice and arrange a variety of colorful fruits in a bowl
for a visually appealing and nutritious breakfast.
Lunch: Vibrant Vegetable Stir-Fry with Tofu

Ingredients:

Mixed colorful bell peppers, thinly sliced
Broccoli florets
Tofu, cubed
Soy sauce, ginger, and garlic for seasoning
2 cups cooked brown rice
Instructions:

Stir-fry bell peppers, broccoli, and tofu in a pan with
soy sauce, ginger, and garlic.
Serve over cooked brown rice for a flavorful and
colorful lunch.

Dinner: Bell Pepper and Black Bean Stuffed Sweet
Potato

Ingredients:

Sweet potatoes, baked
Black beans, cooked
Colorful bell peppers, diced
Cumin, paprika, and lime for seasoning
Instructions:

Mix black beans, diced bell peppers, and seasonings.
Stuff the baked sweet potatoes and squeeze lime
juice on top before serving.
Day 5: Herb Infusion
Breakfast: Basil and Tomato Toast

Ingredients:

Whole-grain bread
Fresh basil leaves
Sliced tomatoes
Olive oil for drizzling
Instructions:

Toast whole-grain bread and top with fresh basil
leaves and sliced tomatoes.
Drizzle with olive oil for a simple and flavorful
breakfast.
Lunch: Quinoa Tabbouleh with Fresh Herbs

Ingredients:

1 cup quinoa, cooked
Fresh parsley, mint, and cilantro, chopped
Cherry tomatoes, diced
Lemon juice and olive oil for dressing
Instructions:

Mix cooked quinoa with fresh herbs and diced cherry
tomatoes.
Dress with lemon juice and olive oil for a refreshing
tabbouleh.
Dinner: Rosemary-Infused White Bean and Vegetable
Casserole

Ingredients:

Cannellini beans, cooked
Assorted vegetables (zucchini, cherry tomatoes, bell
peppers)
Rosemary, minced
Garlic, minced
Vegetable broth
Instructions:

Combine beans, vegetables, rosemary, and garlic in a
casserole dish.
Pour vegetable broth over the mixture and bake until
vegetables are tender.
Day 6: Omega-3 Richness
Breakfast: Flaxseed and Berry Smoothie

Ingredients:

1 tablespoon flaxseeds

Mixed berries (strawberries, blueberries, raspberries)
Almond milk
Instructions:

Blend flaxseeds, mixed berries, and almond milk for a
nutrient-packed smoothie.
Lunch: Walnut and Spinach Salad with Avocado

Ingredients:

Fresh spinach leaves
Walnuts, chopped
Avocado, sliced
Balsamic vinaigrette
Instructions:

Toss fresh spinach with chopped walnuts and sliced
avocado.
Drizzle with balsamic vinaigrette for a satisfying lunch.
Dinner: Chia-Crusted Baked Salmon Alternative with
Roasted Asparagus

Ingredients:

Chia seeds
Salmon alternative (such as marinated tofu or
tempeh)
Asparagus spears
Olive oil for roasting
Instructions:

Coat salmon alternative with chia seeds and bake
until crispy.

Roast asparagus with olive oil until tender.
Day 7: Turmeric Finale
Breakfast: Turmeric-Infused Golden Milk

Ingredients:

Turmeric powder
Almond milk
Maple syrup or honey for sweetness
Instructions:

Warm almond milk with turmeric powder.
Sweeten with maple syrup or honey for a comforting
and anti-inflammatory golden milk.
Lunch: Lentil and Turmeric Soup

Ingredients:

Red lentils, rinsed
Turmeric, cumin, and coriander
Carrots, celery, and onion, diced
Vegetable broth
Instructions:

Cook red lentils with diced vegetables and
turmeric-infused broth.
Season with cumin and coriander for a hearty and
flavorful soup.
Dinner: Turmeric-Spiced Cauliflower and Chickpea
Curry

Ingredients:

Cauliflower, chopped
Chickpeas, cooked
Coconut milk
Turmeric, curry spices
Basmati rice
Instructions:

Simmer cauliflower and chickpeas in coconut milk
with turmeric and curry spices.
Serve over cooked basmati rice for a delicious and
anti-inflammatory curry.
This comprehensive one-week kickstart plan provides
a variety of plant-based meals, rich in cancer-fighting
nutrients and flavors. Feel free to adapt the recipes
based on personal preferences, and consult with a
healthcare professional before making significant
dietary changes, especially for individuals undergoing
cancer treatment. Enjoy the journey towards a vibrant
and healthful plant-based Lifestyles

- ○ **Simple and Quick Weeknight Dinners**

Certainly! A cancer-conscious diet often emphasizes
nutrient-dense, whole foods. Here are two simple and
quick weeknight dinner recipes that align with a
cancer-friendly diet:

Recipe 1: Grilled Salmon with Quinoa and Roasted
Vegetables
Ingredients:

4 salmon fillets
1 cup quinoa
2 cups mixed vegetables (broccoli, carrots, bell peppers)
Olive oil
Lemon juice
Salt and pepper to taste
Instructions:
Preheat the grill.
Salmon fillets should be seasoned with salt, pepper, and a little olive oil.
Grill salmon for about 4-5 minutes per side, or until it flakes easily with a fork.
While grilling, cook quinoa according to package instructions.
Toss mixed vegetables with olive oil, salt, and pepper. Roast in the oven at 400°F (200°C) for 15-20 minutes.
Plate quinoa, top with grilled salmon, and serve with roasted vegetables. Squeeze fresh lemon juice over the dish before serving.
Recipe 2: Vegetable Stir-Fry with Brown Rice
Ingredients:
2 cups mixed vegetables (broccoli, snap peas, mushrooms, carrots)
1 cup tofu, cubed
1 cup brown rice
2 tablespoons low-sodium soy sauce
1 tablespoon sesame oil
Garlic and ginger, minced
Green onions for garnish
Instructions:
Cook brown rice according to package instructions.

In a wok or large skillet, sauté minced garlic and ginger in sesame oil until fragrant.
Add tofu and stir-fry until golden brown.
Add mixed vegetables and continue stir-frying until they are crisp-tender.
Pour in low-sodium soy sauce, toss to combine, and cook for an additional 2-3 minutes.
Serve the stir-fry over cooked brown rice, garnished with chopped green onions.
Remember to consult with a healthcare professional or a nutritionist for personalized advice based on specific dietary needs and health conditions.

- ○ **Celebration Feast for Special Occasions**

Celebrating special occasions with a sumptuous feast is a cherished tradition, and for those on a cancer-healing journey, it's an opportunity to create a menu that not only delights the taste buds but also supports overall well-being. Tailoring a celebration feast to align with a cancer-conscious diet involves careful consideration of ingredients known for their anti-inflammatory and nutrient-rich properties. Here's a detailed guide, along with two recipes, to help you craft a celebration feast that nourishes both body and spirit.

The Principles of a Cancer-Conscious Celebration Feast
A cancer-conscious diet emphasizes whole, unprocessed foods that are high in antioxidants,

vitamins, and minerals. The goal is to reduce inflammation, support the immune system, and provide essential nutrients for healing. Incorporating a variety of colorful fruits and vegetables, lean proteins, whole grains, and healthy fats forms the foundation of a cancer-conscious celebration feast.

Recipe 1: Roasted Turmeric-Ginger Chicken with Quinoa and Berry Salad
Ingredients:
1 whole organic chicken
1 tablespoon turmeric powder
1 tablespoon grated fresh ginger
2 cups quinoa
Mixed berries (strawberries, blueberries, raspberries)
Spinach leaves
Olive oil
Balsamic vinegar
Salt and pepper to taste
Instructions:
Preheat the oven to 375°F (190°C).
Mix turmeric powder, grated ginger, olive oil, salt, and pepper to form a paste.
Rub the chicken with the turmeric-ginger paste, ensuring it's evenly coated.
Bake the chicken for one and a half to two hours, or until the internal temperature reaches 165°F (74°C), in the preheated oven.
While the chicken is roasting, cook quinoa according to package instructions.
In a large bowl, combine cooked quinoa, mixed berries, and spinach leaves.

Drizzle with olive oil and balsamic vinegar, toss gently, and season with salt and pepper to taste.

Once the chicken is done, let it rest for a few minutes before carving. Serve the turmeric-ginger chicken alongside the quinoa and berry salad.

Recipe 2: Grilled Vegetable and Salmon Skewers with Herbed Quinoa

Ingredients:

4 salmon fillets, cut into cubes

Assorted vegetables (bell peppers, cherry tomatoes, zucchini), cut into chunks

2 cups quinoa

Fresh herbs (parsley, dill, mint), chopped

Lemon zest

Olive oil

Garlic, minced

Salt and pepper to taste

Instructions:

Preheat the grill.

Thread salmon cubes and vegetable chunks onto skewers.

In a bowl, mix olive oil, minced garlic, chopped herbs, lemon zest, salt, and pepper to create a marinade.

Brush the marinade over the skewers and grill for 4-5 minutes per side or until the salmon is cooked.

While grilling, cook quinoa according to package instructions.

In a serving bowl, combine cooked quinoa with additional herbs, olive oil, and lemon zest.

Serve the grilled salmon and vegetable skewers on a bed of herbed quinoa.

Conclusion

Crafting a celebration feast in alignment with a cancer-conscious diet is a testament to the power of nourishing the body through thoughtful food choices. These recipes not only embrace the principles of a cancer-healing diet but also bring joy to the table. Remember to consult with healthcare professionals or nutritionists to ensure that the feast meets individual dietary needs and supports overall well-being. Celebrate special occasions with a feast that not only tantalizes the taste buds but also contributes to a journey of healing and vitality.

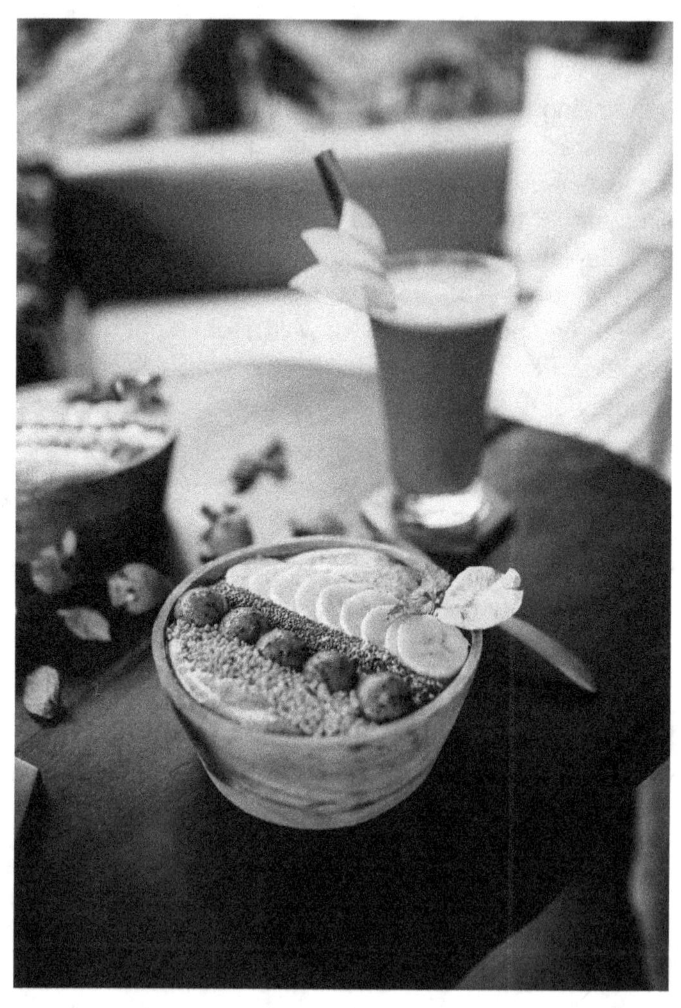

CHAPTER SIX

LIFESTYLE INTEGRATION

○ Mindful Eating Practices

Mindful eating is a practice that encourages a heightened awareness of the present moment, fostering a deep connection between mind and body during meals. When it comes to a cancer diet cookbook, incorporating mindful eating practices can play a crucial role in promoting overall well-being and supporting the body through its challenges. Here's an exploration of mindful eating in the context of a cancer-friendly diet.

Understanding Mindful Eating:
Mindful eating is not just about the food itself; it's a holistic approach that involves paying attention to the sensory aspects of eating, recognizing hunger and fullness cues, and being aware of emotional and environmental triggers that influence eating habits. Applying this philosophy to a cancer diet cookbook involves cultivating a mindful approach to choosing, preparing, and consuming food.

Mindful Choices in a Cancer Diet:
Colorful and Nutrient-Rich Foods:
Start with vibrant, colorful fruits and vegetables rich in antioxidants, vitamins, and minerals. These foods contribute to overall health and can be a flavorful addition to cancer-friendly recipes.

Whole Grains:
Place a focus on whole grains such as oats, brown rice, and quinoa.
These grains provide essential fiber and nutrients while offering a satisfying texture to meals.

Lean Proteins:
Choose lean protein sources including beans, fish, chicken, and tofu.
These choices provide the necessary building blocks for the body without excessive saturated fats.

Healthy Fats:
Incorporate foods high in healthful fats, such almonds, avocados, and olive oil.
These fats offer sustained energy and support various bodily functions.

Mindful Portion Control:
Practice portion control to ensure a balanced intake of nutrients. Mindful eating encourages savoring each bite and recognizing the body's signals of satisfaction.

Mindful Preparation Techniques:
Conscious Cooking:
Engage in the process of cooking with awareness. Pay attention to the colors, textures, and aromas of ingredients. Cooking mindfully can enhance the overall dining experience.

Gratitude Practice:

Develop a sense of gratitude for the nourishing properties of the food. Consider the journey from farm to table and appreciate the effort involved in bringing wholesome ingredients to your plate.

Slow and Steady:
Adopt a slower pace during meal preparation and consumption. This allows for a more profound connection with the food and promotes better digestion.

Mindful Eating During Meals:
Sensory Exploration:
Pause for a minute to enjoy your meal's presentation. Notice the textures and aromas, and savor each bite slowly, engaging your senses fully.

Chew Mindfully:
Chew your food thoroughly, allowing your body to better absorb nutrients and aiding in digestion. This practice also helps in recognizing when you're truly satisfied.

Eliminate Distractions:
Turn off electronic devices, and create a quiet, focused environment during meals. This minimizes external distractions and allows you to be present with your food.

Listen to Your Body:
Observe the indications of hunger and fullness your body sends you.

Mindful eating involves attuning to your body's needs rather than following external cues.

Emotional Awareness:
Be mindful of emotional triggers that may influence eating habits. Cultivate awareness of the relationship between emotions and food, fostering a healthier balance.

Conclusion:
In the context of a cancer diet cookbook, mindful eating becomes a powerful tool for enhancing the overall experience of nourishment. By incorporating mindfulness into food choices, preparation, and consumption, individuals can foster a positive relationship with their meals, supporting both physical and emotional well-being. This approach aligns with the principles of a cancer-friendly diet, emphasizing nutrient-dense foods and mindful practices that contribute to overall health and resilience. As you embark on this journey, savor each moment, appreciating the nourishment that mindful eating brings to your body and soul.

- ○ Incorporating Exercise into Your Routine

Incorporating exercise into your routine is a vital component of a holistic approach to cancer care. Physical activity has been shown to offer numerous benefits for individuals undergoing cancer treatment and survivors alike. From improving overall well-being to reducing the risk of recurrence, exercise plays a crucial role in supporting the body and mind throughout the cancer journey. Here's a comprehensive exploration of how to effectively integrate exercise into your routine within the context of cancer.

Understanding the Benefits:
Enhanced Physical Well-being:
Regular exercise contributes to improved physical health by enhancing cardiovascular function, boosting immunity, and promoting overall strength. This is particularly crucial during cancer treatment, where maintaining physical well-being can aid in managing treatment side effects.

Reduced Fatigue:
Cancer and its treatments often lead to fatigue. Surprisingly, incorporating exercise into your routine can counteract fatigue and boost energy levels. Engaging in physical activity helps improve sleep quality and combats the lethargy associated with cancer treatments.

Mental Health Benefits:
Exercise has profound effects on mental health, reducing symptoms of anxiety and depression. It releases endorphins, the body's natural mood lifters, providing a positive impact on mental well-being during the challenges of cancer treatment.

Improved Quality of Life:

Regular physical activity contributes to an overall better quality of life. It enhances mobility, promotes independence, and fosters a sense of accomplishment, crucial elements for individuals navigating the complexities of cancer treatment.

Tailoring Exercise to Individual Needs:
Consult with Healthcare Professionals:
Before starting any exercise program, it's imperative to consult with your healthcare team. They can provide personalized recommendations based on your specific health status, treatment plan, and individual needs.

Gradual Progression:
Start slowly and gradually increase the intensity and duration of your exercise routine. This incremental approach helps the body adapt and minimizes the risk of injury, especially if you're recovering from surgery or dealing with treatment-related side effects.

Choose Enjoyable Activities:
Opt for exercises that you enjoy, as this increases the likelihood of adherence to your routine. Whether it's walking, swimming, yoga, or strength training, find activities that bring you satisfaction and a sense of accomplishment.

Tailoring Exercise to Treatment Phases:
During Treatment:
Adapt your exercise routine to accommodate the side effects of treatment. For instance, on days when energy levels are low, consider gentler activities like

walking or yoga. Listen to your body and modify your routine accordingly.

Post-Treatment:
As you transition to the post-treatment phase, gradually reintroduce more vigorous activities. Focus on rebuilding strength, flexibility, and endurance. Regular exercise can aid in regaining a sense of normalcy and empowerment.

Social Support and Accountability:
Join Supportive Communities:
Consider joining support groups or exercise classes specifically designed for individuals affected by cancer. Being part of a supportive community provides encouragement, motivation, and a sense of camaraderie.

Buddy System:
Exercise with a friend or family member. Having a workout buddy not only makes exercise more enjoyable but also adds an element of accountability, making it more likely that you'll stick to your routine.

Safety Considerations:
Hydration and Nutrition:
Stay well-hydrated and maintain a balanced diet to support your body's increased energy needs. Proper nutrition plays a pivotal role in optimizing the benefits of exercise.

Listen to Your Body:
Observe how your body reacts to physical activity.

If you experience pain, dizziness, or unusual discomfort, consult your healthcare team promptly. It's crucial to strike a balance between pushing your limits and respecting your body's signals.

Building a Sustainable Routine:
Consistency is Key:
Aim for consistency rather than intensity. Regular, moderate exercise is often more sustainable and beneficial in the long run than sporadic intense workouts.

Set Realistic Goals:
Establish achievable goals based on your individual capabilities. Whether it's a daily walk or a weekly fitness class, setting realistic goals ensures a sense of accomplishment without undue pressure.

Conclusion:
Incorporating exercise into your routine during and after cancer treatment is a powerful way to enhance your overall well-being. It not only contributes to physical health but also plays a pivotal role in mental and emotional resilience. By tailoring your exercise routine to your individual needs, seeking social support, and prioritizing safety, you can embark on a journey that not only supports your body but also empowers you on your path to recovery. Remember, it's never too late to start, and every step, no matter how small, contributes to your overall health and vitality.

CHAPTER SEVEN

TOOLS AND TIPS FOR SUCCESS

- Essential Kitchen Equipment
- Creating a plant-based cancer diet cookbook involves not only selecting the right ingredients but also having the essential kitchen equipment to make the cooking process efficient and enjoyable. From preparing nutritious meals to experimenting with plant-based flavors, the right tools can make a significant difference. Here's a comprehensive guide to essential kitchen equipment for a plant-based cancer diet cookbook, along with their uses.

1. High-Quality Blender:
A high-powered blender is a cornerstone for plant-based cooking. It's versatile and essential for creating smoothies, soups, sauces, and creamy plant-based dishes. Blending helps break down fibers in fruits and vegetables, making nutrients more accessible for absorption.

2. Food Processor:
A food processor is invaluable for chopping, slicing, and shredding a variety of vegetables, nuts, and seeds. It simplifies the process of creating plant-based staples like nut-based crusts, energy balls, and finely chopped veggies for salads or stir-fries.

3. Quality Knife Set:
A sharp and high-quality knife set is fundamental for precise and efficient cutting of fruits, vegetables, and herbs. Investing in good knives not only makes your cooking experience smoother but also ensures safety in the kitchen.

4. Steamer Basket:
Steaming is a gentle cooking method that helps retain the nutritional value of vegetables. A steamer basket is perfect for preparing a variety of plant-based ingredients, from broccoli and cauliflower to leafy greens and root vegetables.

5. Cast Iron Skillet:

A durable and versatile cast iron skillet is excellent for sautéing vegetables, making plant-based stir-fries, and even baking. It adds a depth of flavor to dishes and can go from stovetop to oven seamlessly.

6. Non-Stick Baking Sheets:
Baking sheets are essential for roasting a medley of vegetables or preparing plant-based snacks like kale chips. Opt for non-stick sheets to minimize the need for excessive oil.

7. Spiralizer:
A spiralizer is a fun tool that turns vegetables like zucchini, carrots, and sweet potatoes into noodle-like shapes. It's perfect for creating plant-based alternatives to traditional pasta dishes.

8. Large Salad Bowl:
A spacious salad bowl is crucial for mixing and serving hearty plant-based salads. It allows for easy tossing of greens, grains, and various toppings, making it a centerpiece for nutrient-packed meals.

9. Mandoline Slicer:
Precision in slicing is essential for consistent cooking. A mandoline slicer is a handy tool for achieving uniform slices of fruits and vegetables, facilitating even cooking and presentation.

10. Nut Milk Bag:

For those exploring homemade plant-based milk options, a nut milk bag is indispensable. It helps strain and extract liquids from nuts and seeds, facilitating the preparation of almond, cashew, or oat milk.

11. Herb Mill or Mincer:
Fresh herbs add vibrant flavors to plant-based dishes. A herb mill or mincer allows for easy chopping of herbs, enhancing the taste of salads, dressings, and various recipes.

12. Vegetable Peeler:
A reliable vegetable peeler is essential for removing the skin from fruits and vegetables. It's particularly handy for recipes where the skin might affect the texture or taste.

13. Collapsible Steamer Basket:
A collapsible steamer basket is space-saving and fits into various pot sizes. It's ideal for steaming larger quantities of vegetables, making meal preparation more efficient.

14. Citrus Juicer:
Fresh citrus juice adds zing to many plant-based recipes. A citrus juicer simplifies the process of extracting juice from lemons, limes, or oranges.

15. Glass Storage Containers:
Investing in high-quality glass storage containers is essential for keeping prepared plant-based meals fresh. They are eco-friendly, durable, and allow for easy reheating.

16. Digital Food Scale:
A digital food scale ensures accuracy in measuring ingredients, particularly when following plant-based recipes that require precise quantities for optimal results.

17. Fine Mesh Strainer:
Straining liquids is often necessary in plant-based cooking, especially when making sauces or soups. A fine mesh strainer helps achieve a smooth consistency.

18. Herb Scissors:
Herb scissors make quick work of chopping fresh herbs directly into your dishes, adding bursts of flavor without the need for a cutting board.

19. Vegetable Brush:
A vegetable brush is useful for cleaning and scrubbing fruits and vegetables thoroughly, ensuring they are free from pesticides or dirt.

Conclusion:

Equipping your kitchen with these essential tools sets the stage for a seamless and enjoyable plant-based cooking experience. Whether you're creating vibrant salads, hearty soups, or innovative plant-based entrees, having the right kitchen equipment enhances efficiency and expands your culinary possibilities. As you embark on your plant-based cancer diet journey, invest in these tools to make the preparation of nourishing, flavorful meals an integral part of your Lifestyle

o   **Batch Cooking for Busy Days**

Batch cooking for busy days on a plant-based cancer diet is a practical and efficient way to ensure you maintain a nutritious and wholesome lifestyle while managing a hectic schedule. Adopting a plant-based approach to your meals can offer various health benefits, including reduced cancer risk, as plant-based diets are often rich in antioxidants, vitamins, and minerals. Here's a comprehensive guide to batch cooking for busy days with a focus on a plant-based cancer diet.

**1. ** Meal Planning:

Start by planning your meals for the week. Identify simple and nutrient-dense recipes that align with a plant-based cancer diet. Include a variety of fruits, vegetables, whole grains, legumes, nuts, and seeds. Plan meals that are easy to prepare in larger quantities, making them suitable for batch cooking.

2. Grocery Shopping:

Make a thorough shopping list according to your food plan. You may prevent making impulsive purchases and maintain attention by doing this. Choose organic and locally sourced produce when possible to maximize the nutritional content of your meals. Prioritize colorful fruits and vegetables, as they are rich in phytochemicals that may have cancer-fighting properties.

3. Batch Cooking Basics:
Invest in high-quality storage containers to keep your batch-cooked meals fresh. Consider batch cooking staples like grains (quinoa, brown rice), legumes (beans, lentils), and roasted vegetables. These can serve as the foundation for various dishes throughout the week.

4. Variety and Balance:
Ensure variety in your batch-cooked meals to prevent monotony and provide a wide range of nutrients. Incorporate different colors, textures, and flavors into your dishes. Include cruciferous vegetables like broccoli and cauliflower, known for their potential cancer-fighting properties.

5. Protein-Rich Options:
Explore plant-based protein sources such as tofu, tempeh, edamame, and plant-based protein powders. Incorporate these into your batch-cooked meals to ensure you meet your protein needs for the day. Protein is essential for maintaining muscle mass and supporting overall health.

6. Healthy Fats:
Include sources of healthy fats in your batch-cooked meals, such as avocados, nuts, seeds, and olive oil. These fats aid in satiety and supply important fatty acids. In order to keep your diet balanced, pay attention to portion proportions.
7. Flavor Boosters:

Enhance the taste of your batch-cooked meals with herbs, spices, and homemade sauces. Experiment with different combinations to keep your meals exciting and flavorful without relying on excessive salt or sugar.

8. Efficient Cooking Techniques:
Optimize your time in the kitchen by using efficient cooking techniques. Consider using a slow cooker, Instant Pot, or sheet pan meals for easy and time-saving preparation. These methods allow you to cook large batches with minimal effort.

9. Portion Control:
Divide your batch-cooked meals into portion-controlled servings. This makes it easier to grab a nutritious meal on busy days without the need for additional preparation. Portion control also helps prevent overeating.

10. Freeze for Convenience:
Make use of your freezer to keep extra food in there.

Label and date each container to track freshness. Having a variety of frozen, pre-cooked meals provides convenience on days when cooking from scratch is not feasible.

In conclusion, batch cooking for busy days on a plant-based cancer diet involves thoughtful planning, diverse ingredient selection, and efficient cooking techniques. By incorporating these strategies into your routine, you can maintain a nourishing and cancer-conscious diet even during the most hectic days. Remember to stay flexible and enjoy the process of preparing wholesome meals that contribute to your overall well-being.

CHAPTER EIGHT

RESOURCES

○ **Recommended Reading**

Understanding cancer and its various aspects is crucial for individuals seeking information, whether they are patients, caregivers, or those interested in prevention and overall health. A wealth of literature covers different facets of cancer, from its biology to coping strategies. Here's a comprehensive list of recommended readings that encompass diverse perspectives on cancer.

1. "The Emperor of All Maladies: A Biography of Cancer" by Siddhartha Mukherjee:
This Pulitzer Prize-winning book provides a historical and scientific overview of cancer. Mukherjee, an oncologist, skillfully weaves together personal narratives, scientific discoveries, and the societal impact of cancer, offering a comprehensive understanding of the disease.

2. "When Breath Becomes Air" by Paul Kalanithi:
This memoir, written by a neurosurgeon diagnosed
with terminal lung cancer, reflects on life, death, and
the meaning of both. Kalanithi's eloquent exploration
of his experiences as a doctor and a patient is deeply
moving and offers insights into the human side of
cancer.

3. "The Gene: An Intimate History" by Siddhartha
Mukherjee:
While not solely focused on cancer, Mukherjee's
exploration of genetics provides valuable insights into
the role of genes in health and disease.
Understanding the genetic basis of cancer is crucial,
and this book offers a broader perspective on
genetics that can be applied to various medical
conditions.
4. According to David Servan-Schreiber, "Anticancer:
A New Way of Life":
 Servan-Schreiber, a physician and cancer survivor,
explores lifestyle changes that can complement
traditional cancer treatments. The book emphasizes
the role of nutrition, stress management, and exercise
in preventing and supporting cancer treatment.

5. "Radical Remission: Surviving Cancer Against All
Odds" by Kelly A. Turner:
Turner explores cases of individuals who experienced
unexpected recoveries from cancer. By studying
these cases, she identifies commonalities in their
approaches, providing hope and alternative
perspectives on cancer treatment.

6. "Being Mortal: Medicine and What Matters in the End" by Atul Gawande:
While not exclusively about cancer, this book by surgeon Atul Gawande delves into the broader topic of end-of-life care. It offers valuable insights into the importance of quality of life, personal choices, and the human side of medical care, which can be particularly relevant for those dealing with cancer.

7. "Cancer: A Beginner's Guide" by Paul Scotting:
For those looking for a concise yet informative introduction to cancer, Scotting's book is a valuable resource. It covers the basics of cancer biology, treatment options, and emerging research in an accessible manner.

8. Mahesh K. Shetty, "Breast Cancer: A Guide to Detection and Multidisciplinary Therapy":Focused on breast cancer, this book provides a comprehensive guide to detection and multidisciplinary treatment approaches. It's a valuable resource for patients, caregivers, and healthcare professionals involved in breast cancer care.

9. "The Truth About Cancer: What You Need to Know about Cancer's History, Treatment, and Prevention" written by Ty M. Bollinger:Bollinger's book takes a critical look at conventional cancer treatments and explores alternative therapies. It provides a well-researched perspective on various aspects of cancer, including its history, treatments, and prevention strategies.

10. "My Sister's Keeper" by Jodi Picoult:
While a work of fiction, this novel explores the ethical and emotional complexities of dealing with cancer within a family. It raises thought-provoking questions about medical decisions, morality, and the impact of illness on relationships.

In conclusion, the recommended readings on cancer cover a broad spectrum, from scientific explorations to personal narratives and practical guides. These books collectively offer a well-rounded understanding of cancer, empowering individuals to make informed decisions, find support, and approach the journey with resilience and knowledge. Whether you are directly affected by cancer or seeking to educate yourself on the topic, these readings provide valuable insights into the multifaceted nature of this challenging diseases

- ○ **Online Communities and Support**

Online communities and support networks play a crucial role in providing comfort, information, and connection for individuals affected by cancer. In the digital age, these platforms offer a space where patients, survivors, caregivers, and healthcare professionals can share experiences, resources, and emotional support. Here's an in-depth exploration of the significance of online communities in the context of cancer.

**1. ** Information Sharing:
Online cancer communities serve as vast repositories of information. Members often share personal experiences with treatments, side effects, and coping strategies. This firsthand knowledge can be invaluable for someone newly diagnosed, offering practical insights that complement medical advice. From treatment options to lifestyle adjustments, the wealth of shared information fosters a sense of empowerment and informed decision-making.

2. Emotional Support:
Cancer can be an isolating experience, and online communities provide a virtual haven where individuals facing similar challenges can connect emotionally. Sharing fears, triumphs, and everyday struggles in a supportive environment helps reduce feelings of loneliness. Emotional support is a cornerstone of these communities, fostering a sense of belonging and understanding that transcends geographical boundaries.

3. Peer-to-Peer Connections:
One of the unique aspects of online cancer communities is the ability to connect with peers who have walked a similar path. Survivor stories inspire hope, and the empathy shared among those who have faced similar diagnoses or treatments can be deeply reassuring. These connections, often facilitated through forums, chat groups, or social media, create a supportive network that understands the nuances of the cancer journey.

4. Caregiver Support:
Cancer doesn't only impact the individual diagnosed;
it affects the entire support network, including
caregivers. Online communities recognize the vital
role caregivers play and provide dedicated spaces for
them to share experiences, seek advice, and navigate
the emotional challenges they face. Caregivers can
connect with others who understand the unique
demands of supporting a loved one through cancer
treatment.

5. Real-Time Communication:
The immediacy of online platforms enables real-time
communication, allowing community members to seek
urgent advice, share updates, or simply vent when
needed. Whether through instant messaging, video
calls, or discussion forums, individuals can find timely
support, fostering a sense of connection during critical
moments in their cancer journey.

6. Expert Guidance:
Many online cancer communities feature contributions
from healthcare professionals, offering expert advice
and clarifications on medical topics. While not a
substitute for personalized medical consultation,
these platforms provide a valuable additional resource
for understanding treatment options, managing side
effects, and staying informed about the latest
advancements in cancer care.

7. Access to Resources:

Online cancer communities often compile and share a wealth of resources, including articles, webinars, and reputable information sources. This curated content covers a spectrum of topics, from practical tips on navigating insurance to emotional well-being and lifestyle adjustments. The collective knowledge within these communities transforms them into comprehensive libraries for individuals seeking guidance.

8. Advocacy and Awareness:
Beyond individual support, online cancer communities contribute to advocacy efforts and raise awareness about specific cancer types. Members often engage in discussions about research advancements, treatment options, and policy issues. This collective advocacy fosters a sense of purpose, as community members work together to raise awareness and improve outcomes for those affected by cancer.

9. Anonymity and Privacy:
The option for anonymity in online cancer communities allows individuals to share their experiences and concerns without revealing their identity. This can be particularly valuable for those who may feel uncomfortable discussing their diagnosis openly or wish to maintain privacy. The freedom to choose when and how much to disclose empowers individuals to engage at their own pace.

10. Long-Term Connections:

Online cancer communities can form enduring bonds among members. Shared experiences create a sense of camaraderie that extends beyond the initial stages of diagnosis and treatment. Members often celebrate milestones together, provide ongoing support during follow-up appointments, and continue to share insights as they transition into survivorship.

In conclusion, online communities and support networks have become integral components of the cancer journey, offering a virtual lifeline to those affected by the disease. Beyond information sharing, these platforms provide emotional support, foster peer connections, and contribute to advocacy efforts. As technology continues to advance, the role of online communities in cancer care is likely to evolve, providing even more opportunities for individuals to connect, learn, and navigate the complexities of their unique cancer journeys.

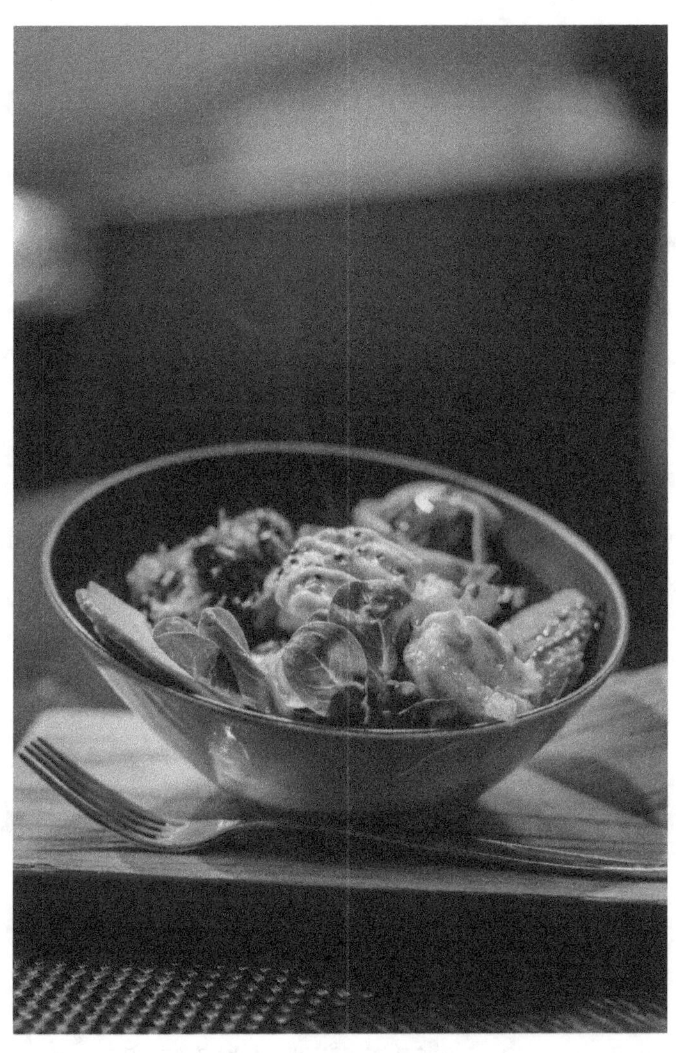

CONCLUSION

Your Journey to Vibrant Health" is not just a cookbook; it's a transformative guide that intertwines the principles of a plant-based diet with the pursuit of overall well-being, especially in the context of cancer. This conclusion encapsulates the details and benefits of the book, inviting readers to embark on a journey toward vibrant health through nourishing, delicious, and purposeful plant-based eating.

1. Understanding the Plant-Based Approach:
At the heart of this cookbook is a profound understanding of the plant-based approach to nutrition. It goes beyond being a mere collection of recipes; it serves as a comprehensive resource, delving into the science behind plant-based diets and their potential impact on cancer prevention and support. Readers are empowered with knowledge, making informed choices that align with their health goals.

2. Culinary Exploration and Variety:
The book takes readers on a culinary exploration, showcasing the vast and vibrant world of plant-based ingredients. From colorful fruits and vegetables to wholesome grains, legumes, nuts, and seeds, each recipe is a celebration of variety. The diverse flavors, textures, and aromas contribute not only to a satisfying dining experience but also to a nutritionally rich and well-balanced diet.

3. Nutrient-Dense Recipes:

Every recipe in the cookbook is crafted with a focus on nutrient density. Ingredients are selected not only for their flavors but also for their potential health benefits. Nutrient-dense meals play a crucial role in supporting overall health, particularly in the context of a plant-based cancer diet. The book emphasizes the inclusion of antioxidants, vitamins, and minerals known for their potential cancer-fighting properties.

4. Practical Batch Cooking Strategies:
Recognizing the demands of busy lifestyles, the cookbook introduces practical batch cooking strategies. The art of preparing meals in larger quantities is demystified, providing readers with efficient ways to incorporate plant-based dishes into their routine even on the most hectic days. Batch cooking becomes a tool for empowerment, ensuring that health-conscious choices are readily accessible.

5. Supporting a Cancer-Conscious Lifestyle:
The recipes presented in the book are carefully curated to align with a cancer-conscious lifestyle. Ingredients are chosen not only for their nutritional value but also for their potential role in cancer prevention and support. Cruciferous vegetables, leafy greens, and plant-based proteins take center stage, offering a palate of flavors while contributing to a holistic approach to well-being.

6. Personalized Meal Planning:
Understanding that each individual's journey is unique, the cookbook guides readers in personalized meal planning. Whether adapting to specific dietary

preferences, addressing nutritional needs during treatment, or simply exploring a plant-based lifestyle for prevention, the book provides a roadmap for tailoring meals to individual requirements.

7. Empowering Through Education:
Beyond the kitchen, the book is a source of empowerment through education. It equips readers with the knowledge to make informed choices about their diet and lifestyle. By understanding the science behind plant-based nutrition and its potential impact on cancer, individuals are empowered to take charge of their health and become active participants in their well-being.

8. Emotional and Psychological Well-Being:
Acknowledging the emotional and psychological aspects of health, the book emphasizes the importance of a positive and mindful approach to eating. It recognizes that well-being is not solely about the nutritional content of meals but also about the joy, connection, and satisfaction derived from the dining experience. The recipes are crafted to nourish not only the body but also the soul.

9. Sustainable and Ethical Eating:
In addition to personal health, the cookbook encourages readers to consider the broader impact of their food choices. It explores the concepts of sustainable and ethical eating, fostering an awareness of the environmental and ethical implications of dietary decisions. This holistic perspective enhances the journey toward vibrant

health by aligning personal well-being with planetary health.

10. Community and Connection:
The book extends beyond the individual, fostering a sense of community and connection. It recognizes that support and shared experiences play a pivotal role in any health journey. Readers are invited to connect with others on a similar path, whether through online platforms, local events, or community initiatives. This sense of belonging amplifies the transformative power of the journey to vibrant health.

In conclusion, "Your Journey to Vibrant Health" is not just a cookbook; it's a guide that intertwines the principles of a plant-based diet with the pursuit of overall well-being. Through understanding, exploration, practical strategies, and a holistic approach, readers are invited to embark on a transformative journey toward vibrant health. This journey is not a destination but a continuous evolution, guided by the principles of nourishment, knowledge, and connection. As individuals embrace the power of plant-based eating, they not only fuel their bodies but also nourish their spirits, fostering a state of vibrant health that resonates in every aspect of their lives

www.ingramcontent.com/pod-product-compliance
Lightning Source LLC
Chambersburg PA
CBHW070901260726
48661CB00004B/1542